LOW PHOSPHORUS COOKBOOK

50+ Smoothies, Dessert and Breakfast recipes designed for Low Phosphorus Diet

TABLE OF CONTENTS

BREAKFAST 6
SEASONED OMELETTE 6
PANCAKES 7
TOAST DELIGHT 8
SEASONED BREAD 9
BAKED CUSTARD 10
SCRAMBLED EGGS 11
MINI WRAPS 12
FRITTATA 13
APPLE TOAST 14
SOFT PRETZELS 15
TUNA SANDWICH 17
BEETS SANDWICH 18
TUNA POCKETS 19
EASY PASTY 21

DESSERTS & SNACKS 24
RASPBERRY MOUSSE 24
SIMPLE BISCUITS 25
BLUEBERRY MUFFINS 26
COOKIE PIE 28
LEMON COOKIES 30
RASPBERRY DELIGHT 31
BLUEBERRY BREAD 33
SIMPLE FUDGE 34
CINNAMON COOKIES 35

SUNDAE ICE CREAM	37
PINEAPPLE PIE	38
HONEY SWEETS	40
SWEET CAKE	42
CREAM CHEESE CUPCAKES	43
CARROT CAKE	44
DONUT CUPCAKES	46
PEACH - RASPBERRY SMOOTHIE	48
CRANBERRY SMOOTHIE	49
WATERMELON SMOOTHIE	50
STRAWBERRY SMOOTHIE	51
BERRY SMOOTHIE	52
PEACHY SMOOTHIE	53
APPLE SMOOTHIE	54
CHERRY-LICIOUS SMOOTHIE	55
CARROT SMOOTHIE	56
PINEAPPLE SMOOTHIE	57
PEAR SMOOTHIE	58
MANGO SMOOTHIE	59
CARDAMON SMOOTHIE	60
GRAPEFRUIT SMOOTHIE	61
ORANGE SMOOTHIE	62
GREEN SMOOTHIE	63
GUAVA SMOOTHIE	64
LIME SMOOTHIE	65
PLUM SMOOTHIE	66

APPLE - CINNAMON SMOOTHIE 67

Copyright 2019 by Noah Jerris - All rights reserved.

This document is geared towards providing exact and reliable information in regards to the topic and issue covered. The publication is sold with the idea that the publisher is not required to render accounting, officially permitted, or otherwise, qualified services. If advice is necessary, legal or professional, a practiced individual in the profession should be ordered.

- From a Declaration of Principles which was accepted and approved equally by a Committee of the American Bar Association and a Committee of Publishers and Associations.

In no way is it legal to reproduce, duplicate, or transmit any part of this document in either electronic means or in printed format. Recording of this publication is strictly prohibited and any storage of this document is not allowed unless with written permission from the publisher. All rights reserved.

The information provided herein is stated to be truthful and consistent, in that any liability, in terms of inattention or otherwise, by any usage or abuse of any policies, processes, or directions contained within is the solitary and utter responsibility of the recipient reader. Under no circumstances will any legal responsibility or blame be held against the publisher for any reparation, damages, or monetary loss due to the information herein, either directly or indirectly.

Respective authors own all copyrights not held by the publisher.

The information herein is offered for informational purposes solely, and is universal as so. The presentation of the information is without contract or any type of guarantee assurance.

The trademarks that are used are without any consent, and the publication of the trademark is without permission or backing by the trademark owner. All trademarks and brands within this book are for clarifying purposes only and are the owned by the owners themselves, not affiliated with this document.

Introduction

Low phosphorus recipes for personal enjoyment but also for family enjoyment. You will love them for sure, for how easy it is to prepare them.

BREAKFAST

SEASONED OMELETTE

Serves: **1**
Prep Time: **10** Minutes
Cook Time: **5** Minutes
Total Time: **15** Minutes

INGREDIENTS

- 1 teaspoon oil
- 1 tablespoon onion
- 2 eggs
- 1 tablespoon water
- ¼ teaspoon basil
- ¼ teaspoon salt

DIRECTIONS

1. In a small bowl beat the eggs
2. Add the water, basil, and salt and stir until combined
3. In a cooking pan, heat the oil and add the onions
4. When the onions turn light brown, pour the egg mixture
5. Cook the omelet for 2-3 minutes on both sides
6. Remove the omelet from the pan and serve

PANCAKES

Serves: **2-4**
Prep Time: **10**   Minutes
Cook Time: **5**   Minutes
Total Time: **15**   Minutes

INGREDIENTS

- ½ cup flour
- 1 egg
- ¼ cup sugar
- ¼ teaspoon baking powder
- ¼ cup milk
- ¼ cup water
- oil

DIRECTIONS

1. In a bowl mix well the flour, egg, sugar and the baking powder
2. Add the milk and water and stir until combined
3. Heat a cooking pan and add some drops of oil
4. Pour some of the mixture in the pan
5. Cook the pancake until it turns brown on each side

TOAST DELIGHT

Serves: 2

Prep Time: **10** Minutes

Cook Time: **5** Minutes

Total Time: **15** Minutes

INGREDIENTS

- 2 eggs
- 1/8 cup milk
- ¼ teaspoon cinnamon
- 2 slices bread
- 1 teaspoon butter

DIRECTIONS

1. Beat the eggs in a bowl
2. Add the milk, cinnamon, and stir until combined
3. In a heated pan toss the butter
4. Soften, on both sides, the slices of bread in the egg mixture and place them in the pan
5. Cook them, on each side, until golden brown

SEASONED BREAD

Serves: **12**

Prep Time: **10** Minutes

Cook Time: **20** Minutes

Total Time: **30** Minutes

INGREDIENTS

- 12 slices bread
- 1 cube butter
- 2 tablespoons onions
- 1 pinch salt
- 1 pinch pepper
- 1 teaspoon basil
- 1 teaspoon oregano
- 1 teaspoon thyme

DIRECTIONS

1. Preheat the oven to 325 F degrees
2. Mix the butter with the onions and spices
3. Spread on top of each slice the butter mixture
4. Place the slices of bread on a baking pan and cook for about 20 minutes

BAKED CUSTARD

Serves: **4-6**

Prep Time: **10** Minutes

Cook Time: **30** Minutes

Total Time: **40** Minutes

INGREDIENTS

- 2 eggs
- ¼ cup milk
- 3 tablespoons sugar
- 1 teaspoon lemon zest

DIRECTIONS

1. **Preheat the oven to 300 F degrees**
2. **Mix the eggs together with the milk, sugar and lemon zest until smooth**
3. **Pour the mixture into a muffin pan**
4. **Place the pan into the oven for 30 minutes or until done**
5. **When ready, let the muffins cool and then remove from the pan**

SCRAMBLED EGGS

Serves: 2
Prep Time: 5 Minutes
Cook Time: 10 Minutes
Total Time: 15 Minutes

INGREDIENTS

- 3 eggs
- ½ cup onion
- ½ cup red pepper
- 1 pinch salt
- 1 tablespoon parsley
- 1 cube butter

DIRECTIONS

1. In a medium bowl beat the eggs
2. Add the onion, pepper, parsley, and salt and stir until combined
3. Heat a cooking pan and melt the butter
4. Cook the eggs by stirring often
5. When ready, remove from pan and serve

MINI WRAPS

Serves: **4**

Prep Time: **10** Minutes

Cook Time: **30** Minutes

Total Time: **40** Minutes

INGREDIENTS

- 2 tortilla
- 4 lettuce leafs
- 10 slices turkey
- 1 cucumber
- 8 slices bacon
- 4 tablespoons mayonnaise

DIRECTIONS

1. Heat a cooking pan and cook the bacon
2. Remove from pan and set aside
3. On each tortilla spread mayonnaise and place the lettuce leaves on top of them
4. Add turkey slices, finely chopped cucumber and the cooked bacon
5. Fold the edges of the tortillas and then roll into a wrap
6. Once rolled, cut them in half and serve

FRITTATA

Serves: **4-6**

Prep Time: **15** Minutes

Cook Time: **15** Minutes

Total Time: **30** Minutes

INGREDIENTS

- 3 eggs
- 1 cup cheese
- 1 tablespoon oil
- 1 onion
- 1 clove garlic
- 2 cups spinach

DIRECTIONS

1. Preheat the oven to 325 F degrees
2. Heat the oil in a cooking pan
3. Add the onion and garlic and mix
4. Add spinach and mix until the leaves become soft
5. In a bowl, beat the eggs together with the cheese
6. Add the egg mixture in the cooking pan
7. Remove the pan and place it into the oven for about 10 – 15 minutes

APPLE TOAST

Serves: 2

Prep Time: 5 Minutes

Cook Time: 10 Minutes

Total Time: 15 Minutes

INGREDIENTS

- 2 eggs
- ½ cup milk
- 2 teaspoons applesauce
- 4 slices bread
- 1 cube butter

DIRECTIONS

1. In a wide bowl beat the eggs
2. Add milk and applesauce and blend until smooth
3. Heat a cooking pan and toss the butter in it
4. Dip the slices of bread in the egg mixture on both sides and place them in the pan
5. Cook on both sides until golden brown
6. When ready, remove from pan and serve

SOFT PRETZELS

Serves: **20-24**

Prep Time: **40** Minutes

Cook Time: **25** Minutes

Total Time: **65** Minutes

INGREDIENTS

- 2 packages yeast
- 4 tablespoons oil
- 5 cups flour
- 8 cups water
- 3 tablespoon baking soda

DIRECTIONS

1. **Preheat the oven to 450 F degrees**
2. **Boil 2 cups of water and dissolve the yeast once the water is warm**
3. **Set aside the dissolved yeast for 10 minutes**
4. **In a medium bowl mix the flour, oil and dissolved yeast until combined**
5. **Cover the dough and set aside for 1 hour**
6. **Start dividing the dough into pieces and shape the pieces into pretzel form**
7. **Set aside for 20 minutes**

8. In a pan, boil the baking soda and the remaining water
9. Dip the pretzels into the boiled water and place them on a greased baking pan
10. Place the baking pan into the oven for 15 minutes
11. When ready, remove the pan and let the pretzels cool for 5 minutes before serving

TUNA SANDWICH

Serves: *1*

Prep Time: *10* Minutes

Cook Time: *30* Minutes

Total Time: *40* Minutes

INGREDIENTS

- 2 slices bread
- ¼ cup tuna
- 2 lettuce leaves

DIRECTIONS

1. Place lettuce leaves on top of one slice of bread
2. Add tuna on the lettuce leaves and close the sandwich

BEETS SANDWICH

Serves: **1**

Prep Time: **10**   Minutes

Cook Time: **5**   Minutes

Total Time: **15**   Minutes

INGREDIENTS

- 2 slices bread
- ½ cup cream cheese
- 1 shredded beet

DIRECTIONS

1. **Spread cream cheese on top of one slice of bread**
2. **Add the shredded beet on cream cheese and close the sandwich**

TUNA POCKETS

Serves: **2-4**

Prep Time: **15** Minutes

Cook Time: **5** Minutes

Total Time: **20** Minutes

INGREDIENTS

- 1 cup lettuce leaves
- ½ cup peppers
- ¼ cup carrots
- ¼ cup celery
- ½ cup broccoli
- ¼ cup onion
- 2 cups tuna
- 4 tablespoons mayonnaise
- 2 pita pockets

DIRECTIONS

1. In a medium bowl mix the lettuce leaves, celery, carrots, broccoli and onions
2. In a separate bowl stir the tuna and the mayonnaise
3. Add the tuna mixture to the vegetable mixture and mix until combined

4. Using a spoon, place the composition into the pockets and serve

EASY PASTY

Serves: **6-8**

Prep Time: **15** Minutes

Cook Time: **40** Minutes

Total Time: **55** Minutes

INGREDIENTS

- 1 packet pastry crust
- 1 cup cheese
- 1 potato
- 1 carrot
- 1 onion
- 2 teaspoons parsley

DIRECTIONS

1. Preheat the oven to 380 F degrees
2. In a pan place the diced vegetables and boil them for about 15 minutes
3. Set aside and let the water drain
4. When ready, using a blender mix for a minute the vegetables
5. Place the vegetable in a bowl and stir together with the cheese
6. Roll and cut the pastry crust in 6 – 8 pieces

7. Place mixture in the middle of the pastry pieces and close them by folding them
8. Using a fork, press on the edges
9. Place them on a baking pan and bake for 30 – 40 minutes or until brown
10. Remove the pan and let cool before serving

DESSERTS & SNACKS

RASPBERRY MOUSSE

Serves: **4-6**

Prep Time: **15** Minutes

Cook Time: **5** Minutes

Total Time: **20** Minutes

INGREDIENTS

- 1 cup whipped topping
- ¾ cup sugar
- 1 teaspoon lemon juice
- 1 cup raspberries
- 1 cup cream cheese

DIRECTIONS

1. In a bowl beat the cream cheese until smooth
2. Add the sugar and lemon juice gradually into the composition
3. Using a fork, crush half of cup of raspberries
4. Mix gently the whipped topping into the composition
5. Add the crushed raspberries and stir until combined
6. When ready, spoon the mixture in glasses and serve

SIMPLE BISCUITS

Serves: **8-10**

Prep Time: **15** Minutes

Cook Time: **20** Minutes

Total Time: **35** Minutes

INGREDIENTS

- 2 cups flour
- 3 teaspoons baking powder
- 2 tablespoon sugar
- ¼ cup milk
- ½ cup water
- 1/2 cup butter

DIRECTIONS

1. Preheat the oven to 325 F degrees
2. In a medium bowl mix the flour, baking powder, and sugar
3. Add the butter and mix well
4. Add the milk and water and stir until combined
5. Start shaping small rolls from the formed dough
6. Place the rolls on a baking pan, previously covered with baking paper
7. Bake the biscuits for 15 – 20 minutes or until brown

BLUEBERRY MUFFINS

Serves: **12**

Prep Time: **15** Minutes

Cook Time: **25** Minutes

Total Time: **40** Minutes

INGREDIENTS

- 1 cup flour
- ½ cup oatmeal
- 2/3 cup sugar
- ½ teaspoon baking soda
- 2 eggs
- ½ cup applesauce
- ¼ cup oil
- 1 lemon
- 1 cup blueberries

DIRECTIONS

1. Preheat the oven to 325 F degrees
2. In a medium bowl mix the flour, oatmeal, sugar, and baking soda
3. In a separate bowl stir the eggs, applesauce, oil and lemon zest

4. Pour the wet ingredients over the dry mix and stir until combined
5. Add the blueberries and mix gently
6. Into a muffin pan pour the composition obtained
7. Bake the muffins for 20 - 25 minutes or until brown
8. When ready, let the muffins cool before serving

COOKIE PIE

Serves: **20**

Prep Time: **20** Minutes

Cook Time: **20** Minutes

Total Time: **40** Minutes

INGREDIENTS

- 3 cups flour
- 1 cup sugar
- 1 teaspoon baking powder
- 1 cup butter
- 3 eggs
- 1 cup jelly
- pinch of cinnamon

DIRECTIONS

1. Preheat the oven to 350 F degrees
2. Mix the flour, sugar and baking powder
3. Add butter and incorporate into the mixture
4. Add the eggs and stir until the composition has the texture of a dough
5. Cut the dough in half
6. Roll one of the balls and place it on a baking pan, arranging the edges

7. Put some jelly on top of it
8. When ready, roll the other half and start cutting strips
9. Place them on top of the jelly layer horizontally or diagonally
10. Sprinkle some sugar and cinnamon
11. Place the baking pan into the oven for about 20 minutes or until the edges turn brown
12. When ready, let the cookie pie cool before cutting and serving

LEMON COOKIES

Serves: **24**

Prep Time: **15** Minutes

Cook Time: **10** Minutes

Total Time: **25** Minutes

INGREDIENTS

- 1 cup butter
- 1 cup sugar
- 1 egg
- 1 teaspoon lemon
- 1 cup flour

DIRECTIONS

1. Preheat the oven to 350 F degrees
2. Mix the butter together with the sugar
3. Add the egg and lemon zest and stir until smooth
4. When ready, add flour and mix until combined
5. Using a spoon, shape mini balls and place them on a baking sheet
6. Cook them for 10 minutes or until brown

RASPBERRY DELIGHT

Serves: *1*

Prep Time: *10* Minutes

Cook Time: *10* Minutes

Total Time: *20* Minutes

INGREDIENTS

- 2 slices bread
- ½ cup ricotta cheese
- ½ cup raspberries
- 1 egg
- 2 tablespoons milk
- 2 tablespoons butter
- oil for frying

DIRECTIONS

1. In a wide bowl beat the egg
2. Add milk and stir
3. On each slice of bread spread ricotta cheese
4. Before closing the sandwich place raspberries on top of one of the slices of bread
5. Dip the sandwich in the mixture, in order to have both sides soften
6. Heat a cooking pan and toss the butter once ready

7. When the butter melted place the sandwich in the cooking pan and cook it, on both sides, until golden brown
8. When ready, remove from pan and serve

BLUEBERRY BREAD

Serves: **6**

Prep Time: **10** Minutes

Cook Time: **15** Minutes

Total Time: **20** Minutes

INGREDIENTS

- ¼ cup blueberries
- ¼ cup water
- 1 teaspoon lemon zest
- ½ cup sugar
- 1 tablespoon butter
- ¼ teaspoon cinnamon
- 3 slices bread

DIRECTIONS

1. Preheat the oven to 400 F degrees
2. Mix all the ingredients, excepting the bread
3. Boil the mixture
4. When ready, pour the mixture into a baking pan
5. Put the bread on top of the composition but not before buttering and sprinkle some sugar and cinnamon on them
6. Cook until the bread turns brown

SIMPLE FUDGE

Serves: *15-20*
Prep Time: *15*   Minutes
Cook Time: *5*   Minutes
Total Time: *20*   Minutes

INGREDIENTS

- 2/3 cup half and half creamer
- 1 cup sugar
- 1 cup marshmallows
- 1 cup chocolate chips

DIRECTIONS

1. Heat a saucepan and add the first 2 ingredients
2. Stir constantly for about 5 minutes
3. When ready, remove the pan and add the marshmallows and chocolate chips
4. Mix until the marshmallows and chocolate chips are melted
5. Pour the composition into a baking pan, previously greased
6. Let the fudge composition completely cool before serving

CINNAMON COOKIES

Serves: ***48-50***
Prep Time: ***10*** Minutes
Cook Time: ***30*** Minutes
Total Time: ***40*** Minutes

INGREDIENTS

- 3 cups flour
- 1 cup sugar
- 2 eggs
- 1 cup butter
- 1 teaspoon baking soda
- 1 teaspoon vanilla extract
- 2 tablespoons cinnamon

DIRECTIONS

1. **Preheat the oven to 380 F degrees**
2. **In a medium bowl mix the flour, sugar, eggs, butter, baking soda, and vanilla extract until the mixture looks like a dough**
3. **Start shaping mini balls of dough and roll them in the cinnamon**
4. **Put the cookies on baking sheet, previously placed on a baking pan**

5. Bake the cookies for 10 minutes or until brown
6. When ready, let them cool before serving

SUNDAE ICE CREAM

Serves: 2

Prep Time: **10** Minutes

Cook Time: **10** Minutes

Total Time: **20** Minutes

INGREDIENTS

- 2 bananas
- 1 cup strawberries

DIRECTIONS

1. Cut the bananas and strawberries and freeze them for about 2 hours
2. Blend them until smooth
3. Place the fruit mixture into bowls and serve

PINEAPPLE PIE

Serves: **6-8**

Prep Time: **20** Minutes

Cook Time: **60** Minutes

Total Time: **80** Minutes

INGREDIENTS

- ½ cup butter
- 1 tablespoon sugar
- ½ cup flour
- 1 crush pineapple puree
- 2 eggs
- ¾ cup sugar
- 3 teaspoons cornstarch

DIRECTIONS

1. **Preheat the oven to 325 F degrees**
2. **In a medium bowl mix the butter together with sugar and flour**
3. **When ready, pour the composition into a baking pan and cook it for 35 – 40 minutes**
4. **In a separate bowl beat the eggs until smooth**
5. **Heat a saucepan and mix, at a low temperature, the pineapple puree with the sugar**

6. Add the cornstarch and stir for 2 – 3 minutes
7. When ready, pour the mixture on top of the eggs and mix until combined
8. Pour the mixture over the baked pie and cook it for another 20 – 25 minutes
9. When ready, let it cool before serving

HONEY SWEETS

Serves: **25-30**

Prep Time: **15** Minutes

Cook Time: **15** Minutes

Total Time: **30** Minutes

INGREDIENTS

- 1 cup shortening
- 1 cup sugar
- 1 egg
- ¼ cup honey
- 2 cups flour
- 2 teaspoons baking soda
- 2 teaspoons ginger
- 1 teaspoon cinnamon

DIRECTIONS

1. Preheat the oven to 300 F degrees
2. In a medium bowl whisk the shortening, egg, and honey
3. In a separate bowl mix the sugar, flour, baking soda, ginger, and cinnamon
4. Stir the dry mix over the wet ingredients until combined

5. Start shaping mini balls and place them on the baking sheet, previously set on a baking pan
6. Sprinkle sugar over the mini balls and bake them for about 10 - 15 minutes or until brown
7. When ready, remove from pan and serve once cool

SWEET CAKE

Serves: **24**

Prep Time: **15** Minutes

Cook Time: **80** Minutes

Total Time: **95** Minutes

INGREDIENTS

- 2 cups butter
- 4 cups sugar
- 2 tablespoons lemon juice
- 6 eggs
- 3 cups flour

DIRECTIONS

1. Preheat the oven to 325 F degrees
2. Using a mixer, blend the butter and add gradually the sugar and lemon juice
3. Add gradually the eggs and mix until each one is combined
4. Add the flour, also gradually and blend well
5. When ready, pour the composition into a greased baking pan and bake it for 60 - 80 minutes or until brown
6. Remove from pan and let it cool before serving

CREAM CHEESE CUPCAKES

Serves: **36-40**

Prep Time: **15** Minutes

Cook Time: **60** Minutes

Total Time: **75** Minutes

INGREDIENTS

- 3 sticks butter
- 225 g cream cheese
- 3 cups sugar
- 8 eggs
- 3 cups flour

DIRECTIONS

1. Preheat the oven to 300 F degrees
2. Blend the butter together with the cream cheese and sugar
3. Add gradually the eggs and mix well after each one
4. Add flour and stir until combined
5. Into a greased muffin pan pour the composition and bake for about 60 minutes or until brown
6. Let the cupcakes cool before serving

CARROT CAKE

Serves: **10-15**

Prep Time: **15** Minutes

Cook Time: **40** Minutes

Total Time: **55** Minutes

INGREDIENTS

- 1 cup sugar
- ½ cup oil
- 2 eggs
- 1 cup carrots
- 2 cups flour
- 2 teaspoon baking soda
- 1 teaspoon baking powder
- 1 teaspoon vanilla
- 2 teaspoons cinnamon

DIRECTIONS

1. **Preheat the oven to 350 F degrees**
2. **Blend the sugar together with the eggs and oil**
3. **Add the shredded carrots and vanilla and mix until combined**
4. **In a separate bowl mix the flour, baking soda, baking powder, and cinnamon**

5. Gradually, add the dry mix over the wet ingredients and stir well
6. Pour the composition into a greased baking pan and bake for 30 – 40 minutes or until brown
7. When ready, let it cool before removing from pan and serving

DONUT CUPCAKES

Serves: 12

Prep Time: 15   Minutes

Cook Time: 20   Minutes

Total Time: 35   Minutes

INGREDIENTS

- ¾ cup sugar
- ½ cup butter
- ¾ cup milk
- 1 cup flour
- 1 tablespoon baking powder
- 1 teaspoon vanilla

DIRECTIONS

1. Preheat the oven to 325 F degrees
2. Blend the butter together with the sugar and vanilla
3. Add milk and set aside, not mixing it
4. In a separate bowl mix the flour and baking powder
5. Add the dry mix on top of the wet ingredients and whisk until combined
6. In a greased muffin pan, pour the composition and bake for 20 – 25 minutes or until brown

7. When ready, remove the pan from the oven and let the donut cupcakes cool for few minutes before serving

PEACH - RASPBERRY SMOOTHIE

Serves: 2

Prep Time: 5 Minutes

Cook Time: 5 Minutes

Total Time: 10 Minutes

INGREDIENTS

- 1 cup raspberries
- 1 peach
- ½ cup tofu
- 1 cup almond milk
- 1 banana

DIRECTIONS

1. In a blender place all ingredients and blend until smooth
2. Pour smoothie in glasses and serve

CRANBERRY SMOOTHIE

Serves: **4**

Prep Time: **5** Minutes

Cook Time: **5** Minutes

Total Time: **10** Minutes

INGREDIENTS

- 1 cup cranberry juice
- 1 cup strawberries
- 2 tablespoons lime juice
- ¼ cup sugar
- ice cubes

DIRECTIONS

1. **In a blender place all ingredients and blend until smooth**
2. **Pour smoothie in glasses and serve**

WATERMELON SMOOTHIE

Serves: 2

Prep Time: 5 Minutes

Cook Time: 5 Minutes

Total Time: 10 Minutes

INGREDIENTS

- 2 cups watermelon
- 1 cucumber
- 1 celery stalk
- lemon zest

DIRECTIONS

1. In a blender place all ingredients and blend until smooth
2. Pour smoothie in a glass and serve

STRAWBERRY SMOOTHIE

Serves: 2
Prep Time: 5 Minutes
Cook Time: 5 Minutes
Total Time: 10 Minutes

INGREDIENTS

- ½ cup strawberries
- ½ cup pineapple
- 1 orange
- ½ milk
- ½ cup spinach

DIRECTIONS

1. **In a blender place all ingredients and blend until smooth**
2. **Pour smoothie in a glass and serve**

BERRY SMOOTHIE

Serves: **4**

Prep Time: **5** Minutes

Cook Time: **5** Minutes

Total Time: **10** Minutes

INGREDIENTS

- ½ cup strawberries
- ½ cup blueberries
- ½ cup cranberries
- ½ cup raspberries
- 1 cup milk
- 1 banana
- 3 cubes ice

DIRECTIONS

1. In a blender place all ingredients and blend until smooth
2. Pour smoothie in a glass and serve

PEACHY SMOOTHIE

Serves: *2*

Prep Time: *5* Minutes

Cook Time: *5* Minutes

Total Time: *10* Minutes

INGREDIENTS

- 1 peach
- ½ cup tofu
- 1 tablespoon sugar
- 1 cup milk
- 1 cup raspberries

DIRECTIONS

1. **In a blender place all ingredients and blend until smooth**
2. **Pour smoothie in a glass and serve**

APPLE SMOOTHIE

Serves: **1**

Prep Time: **5** Minutes

Cook Time: **5** Minutes

Total Time: **10** Minutes

INGREDIENTS

- ½ cup banana
- ½ cup yogurt
- ½ cup applesauce
- ½ cup milk

DIRECTIONS

1. In a blender place all ingredients and blend until smooth
2. Pour smoothie in a glass and serve

CHERRY-LICIOUS SMOOTHIE

Serves: 2
Prep Time: 5 Minutes
Cook Time: 5 Minutes
Total Time: 10 Minutes

INGREDIENTS

- ½ cup cherries
- 1 apple
- ½ cup yogurt
- 1 tablespoon agave syrup
- 2 ice cubes

DIRECTIONS

1. Peel the cherries and apple and cut them into small cubes
2. In a blender place all ingredients and blend until smooth
3. Pour smoothie in a glass and serve

CARROT SMOOTHIE

Serves: *2*

Prep Time: *5* Minutes

Cook Time: *5* Minutes

Total Time: *10* Minutes

INGREDIENTS

- 2 apples
- 5 baby carrots
- 1 orange
- 1 cup spinach

DIRECTIONS

1. In a blender place all ingredients and blend until smooth
2. Pour smoothie in a glass and serve

PINEAPPLE SMOOTHIE

Serves: 2
Prep Time: 5 Minutes
Cook Time: 5 Minutes
Total Time: 10 Minutes

INGREDIENTS

- 1 cup pineapple
- 2 cups blueberries
- 1 tablespoon sugar
- ½ cup water

DIRECTIONS

1. **In a blender place all ingredients and blend until smooth**
2. **Pour smoothie in a glass and serve**

PEAR SMOOTHIE

Serves: **2**

Prep Time: **5** Minutes

Cook Time: **5** Minutes

Total Time: **10** Minutes

INGREDIENTS

- 1 banana
- 1 pear
- 1 apple
- 1 cup yogurt
- 2 tablespoons seeds

DIRECTIONS

1. **In a blender place all ingredients and blend until smooth**
2. **Pour smoothie in a glass and serve**

MANGO SMOOTHIE

Serves: *1*
Prep Time: *5* Minutes
Cook Time: *5* Minutes
Total Time: *10* Minutes

INGREDIENTS

- 1 cup mango
- 1 cup pineapple
- 2 cups spinach
- ½ cup water

DIRECTIONS

1. **In a blender place all ingredients and blend until smooth**
2. **Pour smoothie in a glass and serve**

CARDAMON SMOOTHIE

Serves: **1**

Prep Time: **5** Minutes

Cook Time: **5** Minutes

Total Time: **10** Minutes

INGREDIENTS

- ½ cup mango juice
- ½ cup milk
- 1 cup yogurt
- 2 tablespoon sugar
- ¼ teaspoon cardamom

DIRECTIONS

1. **In a blender place all ingredients and blend until smooth**
2. **Pour smoothie in a glass and serve**

GRAPEFRUIT SMOOTHIE

Serves: **1**

Prep Time: **5** Minutes

Cook Time: **5** Minutes

Total Time: **10** Minutes

INGREDIENTS

- 1 cup lettuce leaves
- 1 grapefruit juice
- 1 apple

DIRECTIONS

1. **In a blender place all ingredients and blend until smooth**
2. **Pour smoothie in a glass and serve**

ORANGE SMOOTHIE

Serves: **2**

Prep Time: **5** Minutes

Cook Time: **5** Minutes

Total Time: **10** Minutes

INGREDIENTS

- 2 oranges
- 2 apples
- ½ teaspoon ginger

DIRECTIONS

1. In a blender place all ingredients and blend until smooth
2. Pour smoothie in a glass and serve

GREEN SMOOTHIE

Serves: **2**

Prep Time: **5** Minutes

Cook Time: **5** Minutes

Total Time: **10** Minutes

INGREDIENTS

- 1 cup pineapple
- 1 pear
- 1 cup celery
- lemon juice

DIRECTIONS

1. In a blender place all ingredients and blend until smooth
2. Pour smoothie in a glass and serve

GUAVA SMOOTHIE

Serves: **2**

Prep Time: **5** Minutes

Cook Time: **5** Minutes

Total Time: **10** Minutes

INGREDIENTS

- 1 cup spinach
- 1 apple
- 1 pear
- 1 cup blueberries
- 2 tablespoons lemon juice
- 1 guava

DIRECTIONS

1. In a blender place all ingredients and blend until smooth
2. Pour smoothie in a glass and serve

LIME SMOOTHIE

Serves: *1*

Prep Time: *5* Minutes

Cook Time: *5* Minutes

Total Time: *10* Minutes

INGREDIENTS

- 1 lime
- ¼ cup pineapple
- 1 cup spinach
- 1 cup passion fruit

DIRECTIONS

1. In a blender place all ingredients and blend until smooth
2. Pour smoothie in a glass and serve

PLUM SMOOTHIE

Serves: 2

Prep Time: 5 Minutes

Cook Time: 5 Minutes

Total Time: 10 Minutes

INGREDIENTS

- 4 plums
- 5 strawberries
- 2 oranges
- 2 tablespoons water

DIRECTIONS

1. In a blender place all ingredients and blend until smooth
2. Pour smoothie in a glass and serve

APPLE - CINNAMON SMOOTHIE

Serves: **2**

Prep Time: **5** Minutes

Cook Time: **5** Minutes

Total Time: **10** Minutes

INGREDIENTS

- 4 apples
- 3 tablespoons lemon juice
- 2/3 cup water
- 1 teaspoon sugar
- ¼ teaspoon cinnamon

- 3 ice cubes

DIRECTIONS

1. In a blender place all ingredients and blend until smooth
2. Pour smoothie in a glass and serve

THANK YOU FOR READING THIS BOOK!

Made in the USA
Coppell, TX
03 December 2021